How Can I Know
My Child's Dentition?

HOW CAN I KNOW
MY CHILD'S DENTITION?

GITI SARAMI

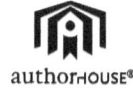

authorHOUSE®

AuthorHouse™
1663 Liberty Drive
Bloomington, IN 47403
www.authorhouse.com
Phone: 1-800-839-8640

Published by AuthorHouse   02/18/2013

ISBN: 978-1-4817-8399-6 (sc)
ISBN: 978-1-4817-8400-9 (e)

Reference: Pediatric and Adolescent Dentistry, MC Donald & Avery

Contents

Introduction

A few words to dear parents

The first appointment to check the oral hygiene and condition should be made within 6-12 months just after the eruption of first primary incisors. Although there is no effective interaction between kids and dentists during this first contact, repeated and successive examinations of the mouth and teeth make the baby fearless and cooperative and the child, thereafter, will have healthy mouth and teeth lifelong.

Chapter 1

EFFECTIVE ROOTS IN PEDIATRIC DENTISTRY

The most important difference between the dental treatment of children and adults is in how relationship is developed and contact is made. In general, when we render treatment to an adult we are in close contact with one person, who is receiving treatment. However, when we provide treatment for a child we have to be in contact with two people, the kid and the parent (mother or father). The parent's, especially the mother's reactions and attitudes are very important for and effective in the child's behavior.

Variables influencing children's dental behavior

A fearful or anxious child who anticipates an unpleasant visit is more likely to exhibit an inappropriate behavior, compared with a child who has a low level of fear or anxiety. Anxiety or fear affects a child's behavior and determines the success of a dental appointment. There are several variables in children's background, which are related to this trait:

A: *Maternal anxiety*

Most investigations reflect a significant correlation between maternal anxiety and a child's behavior during the first dental visit. Although scientific data reveals that children of all ages can be affected by their mothers' anxieties, the effect is greatest with those under 4 years of age.

Therefore, please do not talk about your dental experiences even when your children are in their own room or they are busy with a TV program or other entertainments because they may hear something unpleasant and form a negative attitude toward dentistry. To have positive and cooperative children in dental office, contact your family dentist and ask for help. Never try to explain what dental devices are to your children in your own words.

B: *Medical history*

There is general agreement, however, that children who view medical experiences positively are more likely to be cooperative in the dental office. The emotional quality of past visits, rather than the number of visit, is significant. Pain experienced during previous medical visits is another consideration in a child's history; in fact, parents control their child's thought. If they can control and orient it positively, they can make their children enthusiastic about dental treatment.

C: Awareness about dental problem

Some children may approach their dentists, knowing that they have a dental problem. In this case there is a tendency toward negative behavior during the first dental visit, which might be the result of apprehension transmitted to the child by a parent. This variable highlights the importance of dental visits before dental problems.

Classifying children's cooperative behavior

1. **Cooperative:** Cooperative children are reasonably relaxed. They are good listeners and when guidelines for behavior are established, they perform within the framework provided.

2. **No cooperative ability:** Children with no cooperative ability include very young children with whom communication cannot be established and comprehension cannot be expected. Because of their age, they lack cooperative abilities. Another group of children with no cooperative abilities are those with specific debilitating or disabling conditions. While their treatment is accomplished, immediate major positive behavioral changes cannot be expected.

3. **Potentially cooperative:** The third group of children, who are potentially cooperative, have behavior problems. These children have the capability to behave cooperatively. The child's behavior can be modified and they can turn to cooperative children.

Communicating with children

Communication with a pediatric patient in the dental office, should be established by the dental team only. It is very important for the child to have connection just with the operator; parents' words simply make a child confused and there is no other result but negativity.

Message clarity

In the dental office, sometimes we use euphemisms to make a child enthusiastic to accept treatment. These are like a second language. The following examples are word substitutes that can be used to explain procedures to children.

Dental terminology		*Word substitute*
Rubber dam	⟶	Rubber raincoat
Rubber dam clamp	⟶	Tooth button
Sealant	⟶	Tooth paint
Topical fluoride gel	⟶	Cavity fighter
Air syringe	⟶	Wind gun
Water syringe	⟶	Water gun
Suction	⟶	Vacuum cleaner
High speed	⟶	Mr. noisy
Low speed	⟶	Mrs. Noisy
alginate	⟶	Pudding

Chapter 2

DEVELOPMENT OF THE TEETH

Permanent and primary tooth eruption times are very variable. There is a range of 4-5 months up to 3-3.5 years for the primary dentition to begin erupting and become complete. The exact eruption time can be different from one child to another but all of them have their primary dentition during this period. The sooner the teeth erupt, the sooner they are completed. If there is a deviation from this range, there is possibly a problem which should be consulted with a dentist.

Natal teeth

The prevalence of natal teeth (teeth present at birth) is low. About 85% of natal teeth are lower primary incisors, and only a small percentage has been observed to be supernumerary teeth. Most prematurely erupted teeth (immature type) are hypermobile because of limited root development.

Some teeth may be mobile to the extent that there is danger of dislodgement of the tooth and possible aspiration, in which case the removal of the tooth is indicated. The preferable approach, however, is to leave the tooth in place because they are important in the growth of adjacent teeth.

If you face this situation, please contact your dentist and consult the situation as soon as possible and never act on your own.

Sometimes there is little white or grayish white lesions on the alveolar mucosa which can be recognized as natal teeth. These lesions are usually limited in number, do not grow, and do not need any treatment because they are eliminated without treatment.

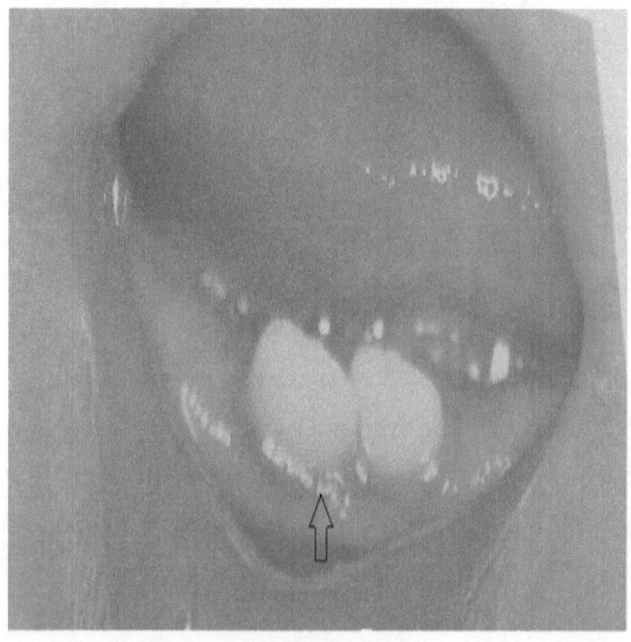

NATAL TEETH

Sequence of eruption of primary teeth

The first primary teeth to erupt are central primary incisors in the lower jaw; these two usually erupt at the same time. The next primary teeth to erupt are lateral incisors followed by first primary molars and the canines. Finally second primary molars erupt. The sequence of eruption in the lower jaw usually (but not always) precedes the upper jaw.

This sequence of eruption is the normal one when there is no problem; however, it is not a hard and fast rule. Sometimes there are variations with no apparent reason, although genetic factors might be involved. This deviation from the normal eruption sequence of primary teeth usually does not result in any problems. The teeth usually erupt on both sides of the jaw at the same time or in a range of maximum ±6 months

Sequence of eruption of permanent teeth

Permanent teeth usually erupt at the age of 5-6. The first mandibular teeth to erupt are first mandibular molars and central incisors. The important thing about the eruption of first molars is that these teeth erupt from the gum pad next to second primary molars and no teeth exfoliate instead. This is very important because most parents do not have any knowledge about it and think they are primary teeth. Therefore, they do not brush and clean them as permanent teeth. Furthermore, these teeth are important from anatomic and position viewpoints. Because of deep undeveloped fissures at the moment of eruption, they are susceptible to decay. In addition, because of their position, in the end corner of mouth next to throat, brushing them is a bit difficult, especially in small children, because brushing can stimulate the gag reflex. Therefore, as soon as their eruption is complete a dental appointment should be arranged to consult with a dentist about preventive measures to avoid decay development.

Soon after central lower incisors and lower molars erupt, lower lateral incisors, upper central incisors and first upper molars erupt, followed by upper lateral incisors. Primary molars and canines are the last primary teeth to be replaced with their permanent successors.

These three teeth (canines, first and second primary molars) in each quarter of the mouth are very important in preserving spaces in the alveolar bone. If these teeth are lost prior to their exfoliation time, some problems can be encountered. Therefore, they should be preserved until they exfoliate normally.

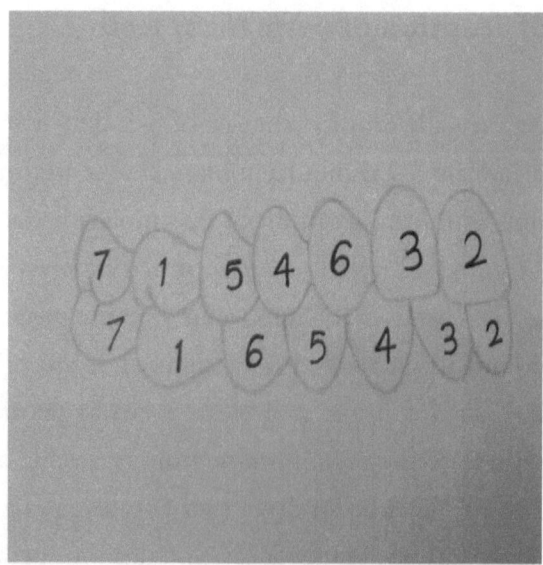

ERUPTION SEQUENCE OF PERMANENT TEETH

What are succedaneous teeth?

You all know about two different kinds of teeth which erupt into the oral cavity.

The first set to erupt from 5-6 months to 2.5-3 years of age is called primary dentition. The second set of teeth which erupt from 5-6 years of age to maximum 13-14 years of age are called permanent dentition. When a baby is born, almost all tooth buds are present in the alveolar bone, and are gradually maturing. Each primary tooth has a permanent tooth under its roots, inside the alveolar bone, which is called a succedaneous tooth. This succedaneous teeth are normally positioned exactly under the roots of primary teeth and when they erupt, make the root(s) of primary teeth resorb (disappear). Finally after they completely erupt into the oral cavity, the primary teeth exfoliate and are replaced by their corresponding permanent teeth.

Therefore, it is very important to retain primary teeth in the oral cavity until permanent teeth beneath them erupt. Thus, primary teeth are as important as permanent ones and should be treated like a permanent tooth if necessary. As it was mentioned previously, permanent molars do not lie under any primary teeth so they erupt directly from the gum pad without exfoliating any teeth. Therefore, most parents do not know they are permanent teeth and therefore, they are susceptible to caries.

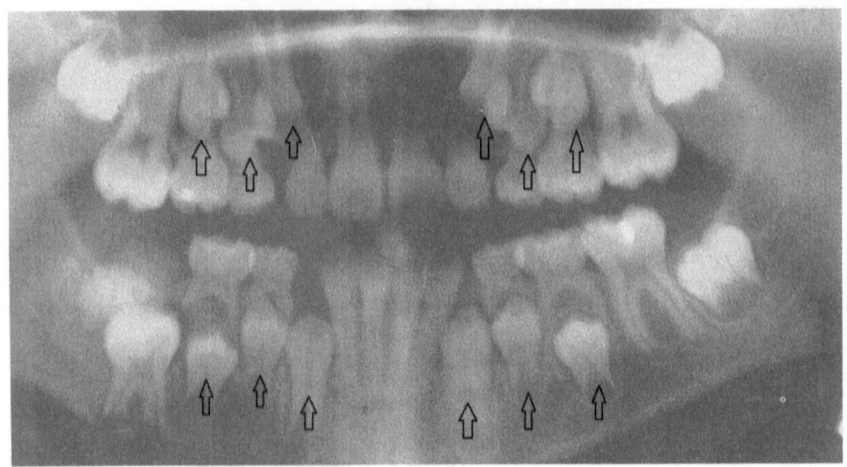

SUCCEDANEOUS TEETH

Lingual eruption of central permanent incisors

It is common for lower central permanent incisors to erupt in the lingual aspect of primary teeth because of a little deviation in their path of eruption. It is a very common cause to worry parents. If the kid with this problem is younger than 7.5 years of age, no problem will be encountered; the primary teeth will exfoliate normally and the permanent teeth will be pushed to place by the force of tongue. However, if the kid is older than 7.5 years of age and primary teeth are not loose enough, they should be extracted because the problem will not be solved by its own.

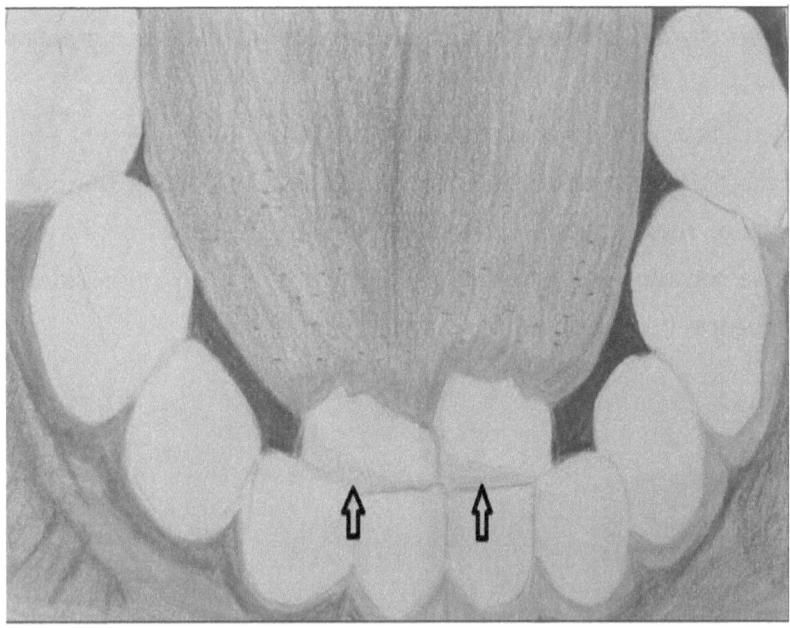

LINGUAL ERUPTION OF CENTRAL PERMANENT INCISORS

Eruption cyst

Sometimes gum pads are hardened and swollen and trauma from the opposing teeth bruise them, worrying the parents because they might be confused with malignancy. After tooth eruption, the problem is resolved and there is nothing to be worried about. If you encounter such a problem, please see your family dentist to have it checked.

What makes a tooth erupt sooner or later than expected?

There are several different diseases which cause tooth to erupt sooner or later than its scheduled time. Therefore, considering the normal range of tooth eruption timetable, which was discussed previously, please consult with your family dentist if you discover considerable differences (a deviation more than 6 months).

Chapter 3

TOOTH ANATOMY

Tooth structure

Both primary and permanent teeth consist of two parts:

1) Crown: The crown is visible in the mouth out of gum pads.
2) Root: The root is located inside gum pads and the alveolar bone and it cannot be seen unless with radiography. This part of the tooth makes it strong and stable in its position because there are lots of periodontal ligaments which attach to root surfaces of the tooth and the alveolar bone, making the tooth strong and flexible.

Contrary to most parents' beliefs, primary teeth, like permanent teeth, have roots and there is no difference in the structure of deciduous teeth and permanent teeth except for their sizes. The two parts of each tooth, crown and root, are composed of three different tissues: enamel, dentin and cementum, which protect the tooth pulp from irritation.

The pulp: The pulp contains vessels and nerves and is surrounded by dentin which has microtubules to transfer nerve impulses by the movement of a fluid inside them. Dentin in the crown of a tooth is covered by enamel which is the hardest and most fragile part of tooth structure and is white and translucent. Dentin in the root section of each tooth is covered by cementum which is not as hard as enamel but is still hard and strong and is mineralized.

Because enamel is fragile it certainly needs dentin as a base to protect it. Dentin is yellow; if enamel is more translucent we can see a yellowish white color on the crown surface.

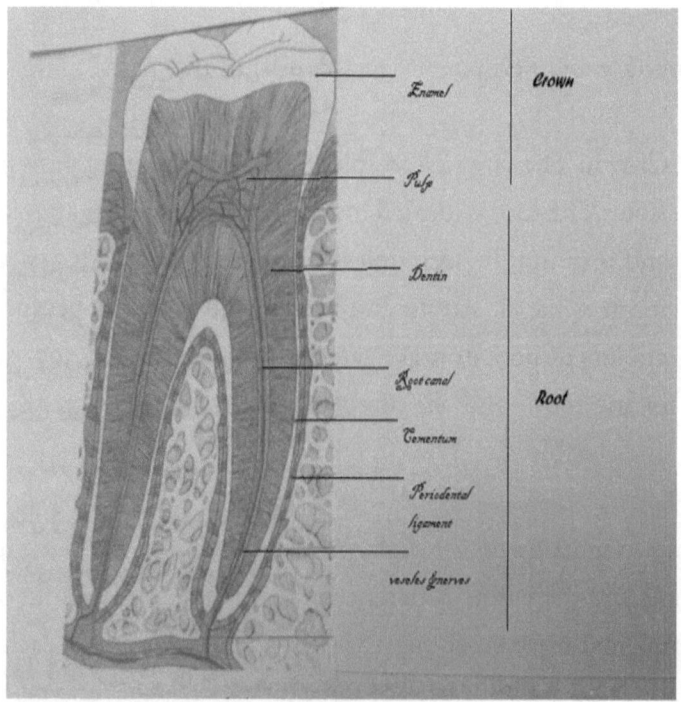

ANATOMY

What is tooth decay and how does a tooth decay?

Specialists believe that tooth decay (dental caries) is an infectious and contagious disease and there are numerous factors involved in its initiation and progression. It is postulated that this disease depends on the host (tooth), food debris and bacteria or microbes which can produce acid. Saliva, substrate and microbes produce dental plaque, which sticks to tooth surfaces. This plaque is produced soon after brushing and gradually grows and becomes thick. If oral hygiene is poor, the oral cavity is the best environment for microbes to produce acid with their substrate. If the environment remains acidic for a long time, the calcified tooth structure will be dissolved. Therefore, brushing and flossing the teeth are very important to maintain good oral hygiene. Tooth decay is a preventable disease and its progress rate is slow at the beginning. If the oral environment is properly controlled, the progression of the decay process can be controlled or even reversed. It is interesting to know that this disease is initiated by a special kind of bacteria and there is a close relationship between the number of the bacteria in the oral cavity of mothers and children. The most common source of transferring this bacterial species to infants or kids is their mothers; therefore, the less number of bacteria in the mother's mouth, the less its counts in the child's mouth.

It is very interesting to know that if a child stays caries-free during primary dentition period, it is possible to stay caries-free during the permanent dentition period, too.

Nursing caries

In recent years it has been recognized that prolonged bottle feeding may result in early dental caries. The clinical appearance of teeth in bottle caries in a child under 5 is typical. There is early caries involvement of maxillary anterior teeth, maxillary and mandibular first primary molars, and mandibular canines. Mandibular incisors are usually unaffected. A discussion with the parents reveals a common factor: the child has been put to bed with a nursing bottle containing milk or a sugar-containing beverage. The child falls asleep, and the milk or sweetened liquid becomes pooled around maxillary anterior teeth, which are good substrates for microorganisms to produce acid, resulting in tooth decay.

The child who falls asleep while nursing, should be made burp and then placed in bed. In addition, parents should start brushing the child's teeth as soon as they erupt and discontinue nursing as soon as the child can drink from a cup at approximately 12 months of age.

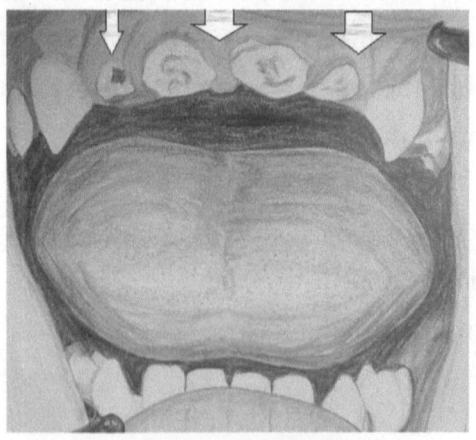

NURSING CARIES

Chapter 4

CAUSES OF TOOTH DECAY

What are the main causes of caries?

1. **Saliva:** It is the main cause of tooth decay; if salivary flow decreases for any reason tooth decay incidence increases. Either its components or its flow and thickness are important in inducing tooth decay. The more and the thin it is, the more the teeth are washed with and the less the decay rate is. However, oral hygiene is still important.

2. **The social and economic status:** Children who are born in poverty are more susceptible to tooth decay than other children and it is more probable for teeth to remain untreated. The incidence of tooth decay among rich families with good economic condition has decreased in permanent dentition, but the incidence of tooth decay in primary dentition in most groups has remained the same as that in the past or even has increased because parents do not know the importance and value of deciduous teeth. The main reason is that parents do

not take care of deciduous teeth but permanent teeth are very important for them.

3. **Anatomic characteristics of teeth:** First permanent molars often have incompletely coalesced pits and fissures that allow the dental plaque to be retained at the base of the defect in contact with exposed dentin because enamel calcification is incomplete at the time of eruption of the teeth and an additional period of about 2 years is required for the calcification process to be completed by exposure to saliva.

The teeth are especially susceptible to decay during the first 2 years after eruption. Other parts of teeth, through which the process of tooth decay can proceed rapidly, are lingual pits on the first permanent molars, buccal pits on the mandibular first permanent molars, and lingual pits on the maxillary incisors.

4. **Arrangement of the teeth in the arch:** Crowded and irregular teeth are not easily cleansed during natural masticatory process. It is difficult for people to clean the mouth properly when the teeth are crowded. This condition may contribute to the problem of tooth decay.

5. **Presence of dental appliances and restorations:** Space maintainers, orthodontic appliances and partial dentures often encourage the retention of food debris and plaque material and have been shown to result in an increase in the bacterial population.

Patients with these appliances should have unusually good oral hygiene. It should be kept in mind that tooth filling materials only replace the destroyed part of the teeth; they cannot prevent tooth decay progression. After filling a decayed tooth, good oral hygiene should still be maintained because tooth decay can happen gradually. Therefore, tooth fillings and restorations should be checked every 5-6 years. Annual dental appointments would be great; if there is a problem, it can be detected and solved easily.

6. **Hereditary factors:** The fact that children acquire their dietary habits, oral hygiene habits, and oral microflora from their parents makes tooth decay more related to nurture than nature. Tooth morphology and enamel defects tend to follow a familial pattern, and therefore heredity may play an indirect role since caries-prone surfaces (anatomically) may be genetically produced.

Diagnosis

Tooth decay can be detected with a dental explorer and light in the dental office.

When you see a brown or yellow discoloration on the tooth surface it is not necessarily tooth decay and in the same manner when your teeth do not have any discoloration it does not mean it is intact.

Sometimes tooth decay starts from tooth contact area; therefore, it is invisible unless examined by radiography. Dental radiographs have a minimum dosage of x-radiation and if a lead apron and a thyroid collar are used, they are safe.

How can tooth decay be prevented?

Regular dental appointments are very important and critical to detect first steps or even beginning of tooth decay processes in order to prevent them.

In order to diagnose a decayed (carious) teeth every dentist needs to examine every single teeth directly and indirectly (by using radiographs). As mentioned previously, dental radiographies have very small x-ray dosages; therefore, they are not harmful.

How can tooth decay be controlled?

Balanced diet, good oral hygiene, patient cooperation and regular dental appointments are very important factors in protecting the teeth. In addition to these factors, preventive procedures can be very effective. It is important not to eat a lot of sweets and sticky toffees or biscuits. In addition, it is advisable to eat on apple or carrot after eating sweets, toffees or chocolates because they have cleaning abilities when chewed. As a result, they can be helpful. Finally, you should brush your kid's teeth thoroughly.

Chapter 5

PREVENTIVE DENTISTRY: BENEFITS AND METHODS

Prevention is better than treatment. Regular dental appointments can make kids more cooperative and obedient. Most people visit a dentist only when they have serious dental problems rather than for checking and controlling their oral health. Accordingly they never care about primary or deciduous teeth because they are temporary. We should know the value and importance of primary dentition in the growth of jaws, development of permanent teeth, and their role in speaking and nutrition of a child. Among primary teeth, primary molars are more important than others because of the following reasons.

Firstly, their exfoliation time is later than other teeth. Secondly, when they are being replaced with their successors, they leave a space in each quadrant of the mouth, which is important in the arrangement of incisors, especially in the lower jaw.

Teeth have a continuous and perpetual growth potential toward the occlusal plane and in the mesial direction; however, because they contact each other at one point or surface, they cannot move easily. Nevertheless, when one or more teeth are not situated in their normal place because of mal-positioning or because of severe damage as a result of decay or even because they have been extracted, the adjacent teeth move into the space, which is not usually in a correct direction. They incline into the space, resulting in a lot of problems, which are difficult to solve.

When there is less information about preventive and pediatric dentistry, parents inadvertently make mistakes and they have to pay a high price to solve these problems. On the other hand, because the majority of oral diseases are not harmful and serious, people pay inadequate attention to them.

Preventive dentistry

There is a frequently asked question: Is tooth decay preventable?

As mentioned previously, there are a lot of factors involved in tooth decay but some, which are more important than others, are presence of decay-inducing (cariogenic) bacteria, an environment or a substrate (sugar, food debris, etc) and poor oral hygiene (brushing, use of dental floss). These are three important and must co-exist to result in tooth decay. There are some protocols to decrease the presence of these agents. Therefore, by following these protocols tooth decay is preventable.

The methods of prevention

1. Preventive operative dentistry (fissure sealant therapy)
2. Preventive orthodontics
3. Fluoride therapy
4. Mechanical procedures of tooth decay control
   a) Manual toothbrush
   b) Powered toothbrush
   c) Dental floss

1) Preventive operative dentistry or fissure sealant therapy

This is a very simple and conservative method to seal pits and fissures of teeth which are prone to caries, specifically within two years after their eruption. In this method a special material is placed in the deepest part of pits and fissures of occlusal surfaces of teeth to protect the teeth against decay.

2) Preventive orthodontics

Sometimes the position of teeth in jaw is conducive to food impaction and poor oral hygiene. Therefore, orthodontic treatment and correction of malposed teeth will pave the way for maintaining good oral hygiene by making it possible to clean teeth properly. Another advantage of preventive orthodontic treatment is the use of space maintainers.

A space maintainer (S.M.) is a simple device (band and loop) which maintains the lost tooth space until the permanent tooth erupts and does not let adjacent teeth move or tilt into the free space. There are different kinds of S.M. and each is built for their advantages. By using S.M we can protect most mal-positionings without orthodontics brackets.

3) Fluoride therapy

Use of fluoride mouth rinses or gels is very important in controlling and preventing tooth decay in both children and adults.

Fluoride can be used in different ways, including fluoride tablets, fluoridated water, fluoridated mouth washes, fluoridated toothpastes and fluoridated gels and solutions. All of these have their own advantages and the choice is made by the dentist. Use of fluoride tablets or fluoridated water supply is specific to cities, where fluoridated water supply is not available. Use of fluoride mouth washes and gels in combination is very useful to strengthen tooth structure. The former is used personally at home and the latter is used in the dental office by the dentist. Using both of them can be more effective than using just one of them. It is recommended that fluoride gel or solution be used every six months for children and adolescents without tooth decay. If there are widespread carious lesions, the dentist will decide how often it should be used. It is important to notice that fluoride is a toxic material and should be used only as recommended by a dentist.

How does fluoride act?

Use of fluoride results in penetration of fluoride into the dentin and enamel of unerupted and erupted teeth, making tooth structure strong enough to resist bacterial acid attack. In addition, fluoride is released into saliva. Although it is less concentrated, it can be useful to reduce release of acid by bacteria and increase enamel strength. On the other hand, fluoride in the saliva can penetrate into newly erupted teeth and increase calcification of enamel and decrease incidence of tooth decay.

Use of fluoridated mouth rinses, solutions, gels and toothpastes topically (on the tooth surface) is as useful as the fluoride tablets and fluoridated water except for the fact that locally used agents cannot penetrate into unerupted tooth structure.

4) Mechanical methods of caries control

a) **Manual toothbrush**

The usual method of cleaning teeth and mouth is the use of toothbrushes. Most toothbrushes which are commercially available have synthetic bristles. This part of a toothbrush is the most important part. Toothbrushes are classified as soft, medium or hard, based on the width of these bristles. A soft brush is preferable in pediatric dentistry because of the decreased incidence of gingival tissue trauma, and its increased interproximal cleaning ability.

The most preferable toothbrush in pediatric dentistry is a toothbrush with a small head and a thick handle so that children can use it much more easily. The most frequently asked question is: *How often should a used toothbrush be replaced with a new one?*

The best recommendation is: *whenever a toothbrush seems completely well-worn.*

b) **Powered toothbrush**

There is a little difference in plaque removal properties between powered or electric toothbrushes and manual ones; however, because it can be interesting for children to use the electric one, it may persuade them to brush their teeth more enthusiastically.

c) **Dental floss**

Although brushing the teeth is the most commonly used method of plaque control or removal, it cannot be the only way of tooth cleaning because it cannot clean interproximal areas. There are several different methods for interproximal cleaning, including interdental brushes, Y-shaped floss holders, disposable floss holders and picks, and wooden toothpicks. Among all of them dental floss is the most frequently used tool. Other methods can be used under special circumstances—in orthodontics or prosthodontics.

Toothpaste

A toothpaste, a combination of different agents, cleans the teeth and gums. Children's toothpaste should have less fluoride, less abrasive effect and A.D.A's confirmation.

Most toothpastes are flavored for cheering up and motivate children. The amount of toothpaste used by/for kids under 9 should be as little as possible, for example the size of a pea or less. For children under 5-6 years of age washing the mouth and teeth with a toothbrush and pure water is recommended because they cannot spit the toothpaste out and may swallow it inadvertently; if they swallow large amounts of fluoride, it can be harmful for them.

The techniques of flossing and brushing

For children under 6 years of age, the most effective and easiest way for brushing is the horizontal scrub method. The brush is placed horizontally on buccal and lingual surfaces and moved back and forth with a scrubbing motion.

Flossing: For flossing, the following method is recommended.

1. A piece of 46-61-cm (18-24 inches) long of dental floss is obtained, and the ends are wrapped around the patient's or parents middle fingers to allow enough floss to be placed between the hands for the thumbs to touch each other when the hands are laid flat.

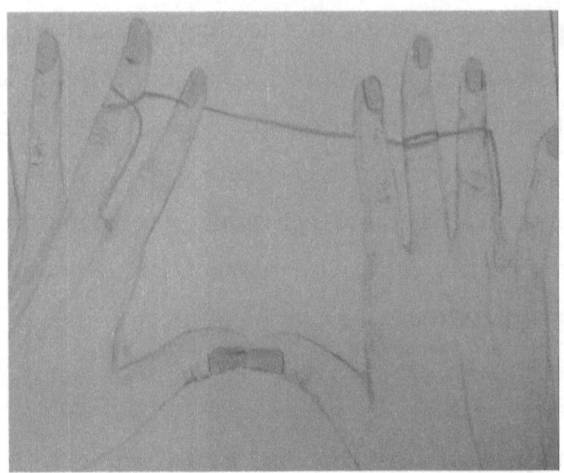

HOW TO FLOSS

2. Using the thumbs and index fingers to guide the floss, it is gently sawed between the two teeth to be cleaned. To avoid gingival trauma, care should be exercised when cleaning interproximal areas.

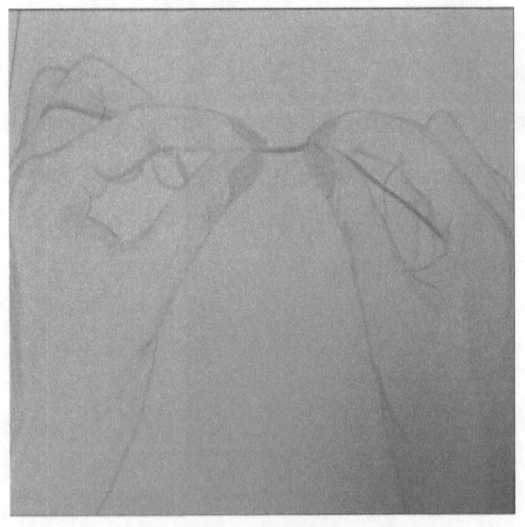

HOW TO FLOSS

3. The floss is then manipulated into a c-shape around each tooth individually and moved in a cervico-occlusal reciprocating motion until the plaque is removed. Between each pair of teeth the floss is repositioned on the fingers so that fresh, unsoiled part of the floss is used at each new location. For children floss with holders can be used because their use is easier than the regular one which needs more practice.

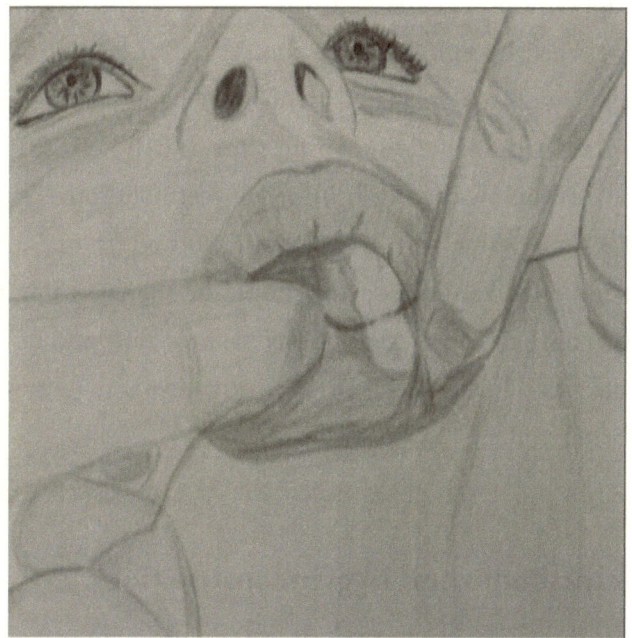

HOW TO FLOSS

Time considerations

How often should patients brush and floss their teeth and for how long?

All oral hygiene practices for children should be carried out under parents' supervision. They should brush their teeth at least once or twice a day. Each brushing session should last at least 1 minute and accomplished with a fluoridated dentifrice, with flossing and other plaque removal activities adding to this time. If children are not able to spit out, it is recommended to brush their teeth without a fluoridated toothpaste. Pure water and a brush will suffice. If oral hygiene is accomplished only once per day, it should be the last thing the child does before going to bed at night. Since salivary flow and its buffering capacity decrease during sleep, it is advantageous to remove plaque before bedtime.

Age-specific home oral hygiene instructions

Infants (0-1 years of age)

It is important to follow a few basic home oral hygiene instructions for the children during their first year of life. It is generally agreed that plaque removal activities should begin upon eruption of the first primary teeth. Some dental practitioners recommend cleaning and massaging of the gums before this to help in establishment of a healthy oral flora and to aid in teething. This early cleaning must be carried out by parents. It can be accomplished by wrapping a moistened piece of gauze around the parents' finger and gently massage the teeth and gingival tissues.

Toddlers (1-3 years of age)

During this period toothbrush is introduced to control and remove plaque if it was not accomplished in the previous age bracket. Because of this age group's inability to expectorate and the possibility of fluoride ingestion, only a small pea-sized amount of toothpaste should be used or only a toothbrush and water are used without any toothpaste.

Most children enjoy brushing their teeth at this age but they cannot remove adequate plaque from their teeth. Therefore, their parents should be the primary caregivers in these procedures. Flossing may be needed if any interproximal contacts are closed. Positioning of the child and parent is an important part in toothbrushing. You had better sit on the floor and place the child's head between your thighs with the child's arms and legs carefully controlled by your legs.

Preschool (3-6 years of age)

Although children in this age range demonstrate significant improvement in their ability to manipulate the toothbrush, it is still the responsibility of the parent to be the primary provider of oral hygiene procedures. If the child shows interest in doing this job by his or her own, let him/her do it; however, finally you should brush their teeth again.

Fluoride ingestion still remains a concern for this age group, so it is important to continue to use of pea-sized toothpaste on child's brush. Proper positioning still is useful for this age group in performing oral hygiene practices.

One method advocated is with the parent standing behind the child, with the parent and child facing the same direction. The child rests his/her head back into the parent's non-dominant arm. This is also appropriate for flossing. It is also during this stage that fluoride gels and rinses might be introduced for home use; however, because of the risk of ingestion it is only recommended to patients who demonstrate a moderate-to-high caries risk.

School age (6-12 years of age)

This stage is marked by acceptance of increasing responsibilities by children, such as assuming their homework and household chores. In this stage parents should supervise instead of actively brushing their children's teeth. During the second half of this stage children can carry out their oral hygiene procedures by their own (brushing and flossing); parents should help them in some difficult-for-reach areas. In this age group there is no risk of ingestion; therefore, children can use fluoride gels and rinses easily.

Adolescents (12-19 years of age)

During this period adolescents can perfectly assume their oral hygiene procedures but because of age-related problems oral hygiene might be complicated by reactions of rebellion against external authority. On

Chapter 6

RESTORATION OR FILLING OF TEETH

Whenever teeth develop caries, there is no choice but to remove the decayed part (decalcified region) and place restorative materials instead. These materials are not permanent and even with a very good oral hygiene and with very high-quality materials and meticulous restorative procedures, after a while (maximum 6-8 years) they need to be checked by a dentist and radiographic inspections because there is the possibility of recurrent caries under the restorative materials due to leakage. These recurrent lesions are closely related with

1. thorough removal of decalcified parts and tissues
2. dental practitioner's professional skills and proficiency
3. quality of filling materials
4. adoption of oral hygiene procedures by the patient.

If there is any failure in any section, recurrent lesions will ensue very soon after filling. There is a very important consideration after tooth decay develops and everyone should realize that dentists remove only the decayed and decalcified part of teeth rather than intact parts. Therefore, since teeth have 5 surfaces, which can develop caries at any time, please pay special attention to this very important aspect. Sometimes patients get confused and do not know which part has become carious.

Local anesthesia

Local anesthesia is a procedure to control pain in most medical fields, especially in dentistry.

In pediatric dentistry, since the majority of children are afraid of needles or syringes dentists try not to show them to children; dentists usually use anesthesia gel before inserting the needle into the area so that children would not feel any pain. In addition, since they cannot see the syringe (in a special method of injection) they can never realize they have received an injection by a needle. Therefore, dentists ask the parents not to talk about this procedure in the presence of their children. Older children can understand and cannot tolerate a little pain, but very young children are afraid of needles and cannot understand the explanation well, so they might get confused. Therefore, it is better not to try to explain why they should have an injection; we can only tell them their teeth and mouths are going to fall asleep for a period of time so we can remove bacteria easily. Trust your dentists and let them do their job as perfectly as they can.

Chapter 7

TRAUMA TO TEETH AND MOUTH

Children, because of their age, are active; so they might fall and injure or wound any part of their body. Among all the body parts, head and neck are more prone to traumatic injuries. Trauma to the oral region can have different consequences, so a little bit of knowledge about different methods of treatment can be helpful for both parents.

During trauma to the face the possibility of its occurrence at maxillary and mandibular central incisors is high, and of these, central maxillary incisors are more susceptible to trauma than others because of their position in the mouth. Trauma can cause different kind of injuries to teeth and we can classify them as follows:

1. **Tooth crown fracture:** This can be classified as the follows:

   A. Fracture of tooth edge: This kind of fracture is not so serious; if it is sharp and can hurt the lips we only need to smooth and polish it.

B. A major part of tooth crown is fractured but the pulp is not involved.

C. The fracture of major part of tooth crown involves the pulp, too.

    As fracture of any size may occur you should see a dentist to consult with.

2. **Displacement of deciduous and permanent teeth:**

    A. **Luxation:** When trauma is not so serious luxation happens. In some cases it is not so serious and no treatment is necessary but sometimes it is serious and the tooth involved should be repositioned, fixed to the adjacent teeth, and followed for a while.

    B. **Extrusion:** The tooth is luxated and comes out of the alveolar socket a little bit. The extrusive luxated and only luxated primary teeth remain luxated until they are replaced by permanent teeth. But the extrusive luxation of permanent teeth usually results in pulpitis. The immediate treatment involves careful repositioning of the tooth and stabilization. The tooth should be followed in recall visits to check for the vitality of pulp within 2-3 weeks.

    C. **Intrusion:** The tooth is luxated or not but it is intruded into the alveolar socket and is below the occlusion or occlusal plane. In such a case a dental x-ray is necessary to check the position of the intruded tooth. If the intruded tooth is a primary tooth, since the developing permanent incisor tooth buds normally lie lingual to the roots of primary central incisors, the primary tooth usually remains labial to the developing permanent tooth. If the primary tooth is found to be lingual to the developing permanent tooth, it should be removed. If the intruded tooth is a permanent tooth we can gradually reposition it by orthodontic procedures within 2-3 weeks and then other treatments can be followed if necessary. It is important to act as fast as possible in any injuries happening in the oral areas. Knowledge about the consequences and prognoses of injuries can help parents decide and act as wisely as possible.

D. **Avulsion:** This mostly happens among young boys. Sometimes trauma causes a tooth to come out of its socket completely. It is very important to act very quickly and clean the tooth gently under running water and then put it in a clean bath of milk or saliva; if none is available, it should be placed in just water and a dentist should be visited within maximum 2 hours. For replanting the tooth if you do not have enough time, just put the tooth in the alveolar socket and go to a clinic. Remember that in this kind of injury time is very important to replant the tooth. After 2 hours the tooth cannot be replanted because of the blood clot forming in the tooth socket.

www.ingramcontent.com/pod-product-compliance
Lightning Source LLC
Chambersburg PA
CBHW030545290526
45786CB00004B/1879